SELF-CARE HEALTH JOURNAL

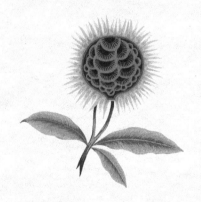

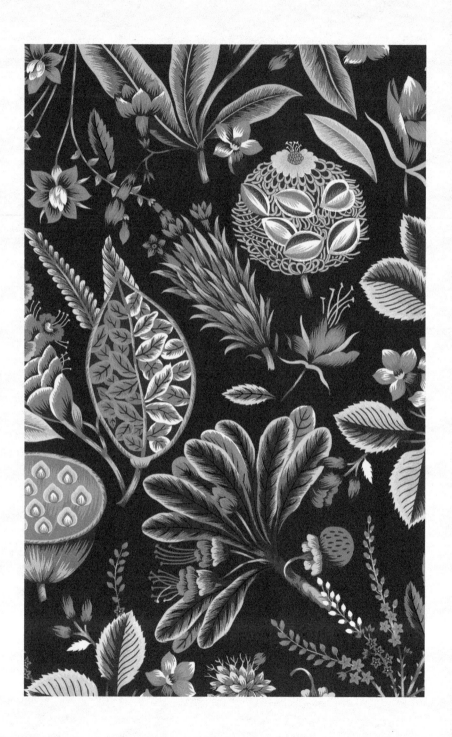

✦ SELF-CARE ✦
Health Journal

A 90-DAY FOOD, FITNESS, AND WELL-BEING TRACKER

ROCKRIDGE
PRESS

Interior and Cover Designer: Lisa Schreiber
Art Producer: Sue Bischofberger
Editor: Rebecca Markley
Production Editor: Ashley Polikoff

Illustration © TSTUDIO/Creative Market
Paper texture © Greta Ivy/Creative Market

ISBN: 978-1-638-78139-4
R0

This book belongs to

_____

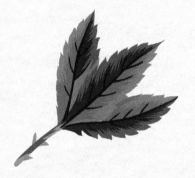

SO, WHAT IS SELF-CARE?

Self-care is taking an active and deliberate role in protecting your physical, mental, and emotional well-being, especially during stressful or challenging times. Wondering where to start? The foundations of self-care include basic needs like sleep, exercise, and nutrition. These are vital to your overall wellness and should always be your first priority. After that, we have work, relationships, time with loved ones, and hobbies. Nourishing these aspects of your life helps prevent stress and burnout. At the top of the pyramid, you'll find all of the "extras"—things that we can add to our lives to reduce our stress burden and keep our tanks topped off. These include meditation, massage, yoga, time in nature, pampering, supplements, laughter, and beyond.

✦ SELF-CARE PYRAMID ✦

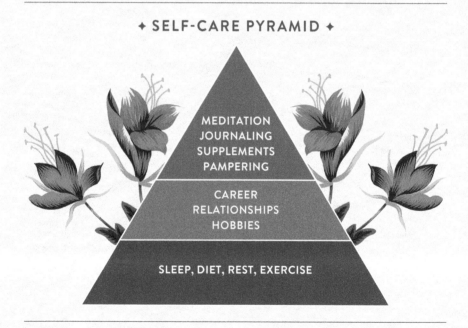

MEDITATION
JOURNALING
SUPPLEMENTS
PAMPERING

CAREER
RELATIONSHIPS
HOBBIES

SLEEP, DIET, REST, EXERCISE

HOW TO USE THIS JOURNAL

Maybe your therapist has suggested that you start practicing more self-care. Or maybe you've made a commitment to yourself to start paying more attention to how you feel. But what does that look like in practice?

The journal pages that follow invite you to track your daily activities, habits, and other practices in service of caring for your mind, body, and spirit. It can be hard to remember what you've done or felt even in the span of just one day, so consider carrying it around with you and jotting notes as you go. Each daily entry includes two pages: the left-hand page prompts you to document activities and feelings that influence your physical well-being, while the right-hand page asks you to track and reflect on your mood.

The right-hand pages also leave space for recording how you've supported your well-being in a variety of other areas: physical, emotional, mental, practical, social, and spiritual. Following are brief descriptions of each area, with suggestions to help you get started or continue on your self-care journey.

PHYSICAL

Physical well-being is not just about preventing illness; it also includes taking steps to feel energized, reduce pain or injury, and feel good physically in general.

SUGGESTIONS: Getting enough sleep, staying hydrated, taking walks after work, taking care of medical needs, taking supplements

EMOTIONAL

Emotional well-being includes any activity that helps you connect, process, and reflect on a range of emotions. Regular practice of these types of activities can help you center yourself or embrace self-care strategies that help you feel good when challenging or stressful situations inevitably arise.

SUGGESTIONS: Seeing a therapist, breath work, meditating, setting boundaries, reflecting on your feelings, journaling, creating art, listening to music

MENTAL

Mental well-being is both about intellectual stimulation and preserving cognitive functions like memory, critical thinking, and the ability to concentrate.

SUGGESTIONS: Taking "brain breaks" during periods of study or concentration, reading a book, solving a puzzle, going to a museum, using your vacation time at work, not working on days off

PRACTICAL

Practical well-being includes habits, tasks, and planning that you need to do to prevent future stressful situations.

SUGGESTIONS: Budgeting, setting up appointments, brushing your teeth, taking professional development classes, organizing your closet, keeping your insurance up-to-date

SOCIAL

Social well-being includes any activity that positively fosters the relationships with people in your life. Maintaining these relationships means both connecting and setting healthy boundaries.

SUGGESTIONS: Having dinner with friends, calling your family, going on a date, seeking help from friends or coworkers when you need it

SPIRITUAL

Spiritual well-being is about nourishing your spirit in any larger way to feel connected with the rest of the world or beyond. Think of it as anything you would do to "feed the soul." Spiritual here doesn't mean religious, but it can be.

SUGGESTIONS: Being in nature, meditating, volunteering, going to a place of worship, dedicating time for self-reflection

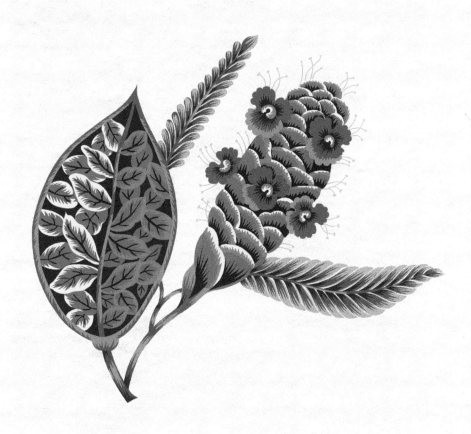

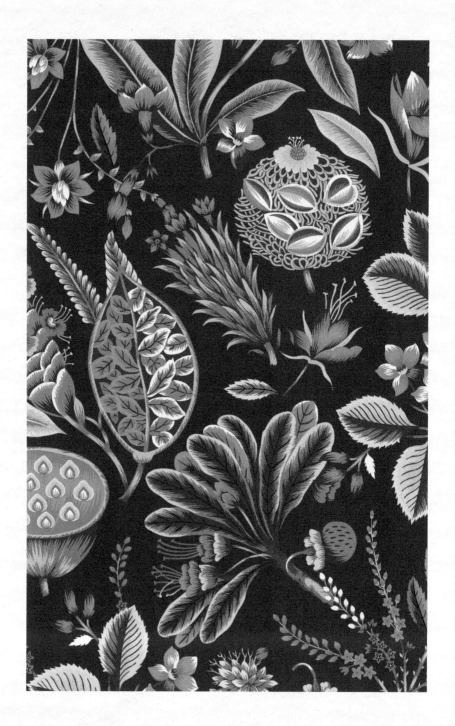

My Intention for This Journal

What are you hoping to get out of this journal? Are there specific areas of self-care that you'd like to improve on?

_____

_____

_____

_____

_____

_____

AN AFFIRMATION TO LOOK BACK ON:

_____

_____

_____

_____

_____

_____

DATE: _____

LAST NIGHT'S SLEEP: _____ HOURS _____ MINUTES

QUALITY: _____

FOOD I ATE

MEAL 1	SNACKS & BEVERAGES

MEAL 2	

MEAL 3	HYDRATION
	🜄 = 10 ounces of water

🜄 🜄 🜄 🜄

🜄 🜄 🜄 🜄

ACTIVITY	NOTES

ENERGY LEVEL	1	2	3	4	5

(1 = very low; 2 = low; 3 = moderate; 4 = high; 5 = very high)

MY MOOD

MORNING: _____

AFTERNOON: _____

EVENING: _____

ON MY MIND TODAY:

HOW I CARED FOR MYSELF TODAY

PHYSICAL: _____

_____

EMOTIONAL: _____

_____

MENTAL: _____

_____

PRACTICAL: _____

_____

SOCIAL: _____

_____

SPIRITUAL: _____

_____

TODAY I'M GRATEFUL FOR:

DATE: _____

LAST NIGHT'S SLEEP: _____ HOURS _____ MINUTES

QUALITY: _____

FOOD I ATE

MEAL 1

MEAL 2

MEAL 3

SNACKS & BEVERAGES

HYDRATION

◊ = 10 ounces of water

◊ ◊ ◊ ◊

◊ ◊ ◊ ◊

ACTIVITY

NOTES

ENERGY LEVEL 1 2 3 4 5

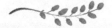

(1 = very low; 2 = low; 3 = moderate; 4 = high; 5 = very high)

MY MOOD

MORNING: _____

AFTERNOON: _____

EVENING: _____

ON MY MIND TODAY:

HOW I CARED FOR MYSELF TODAY

PHYSICAL: _____

_____

EMOTIONAL: _____

_____

MENTAL: _____

_____

PRACTICAL: _____

_____

SOCIAL: _____

_____

SPIRITUAL: _____

_____

TODAY I'M GRATEFUL FOR:

DATE: _____

LAST NIGHT'S SLEEP: _____ HOURS _____ MINUTES

QUALITY: _____

FOOD I ATE

MEAL 1

MEAL 2

MEAL 3

SNACKS & BEVERAGES

HYDRATION

◊ = 10 ounces of water

◊ ◊ ◊ ◊

◊ ◊ ◊ ◊

ACTIVITY

NOTES

ENERGY LEVEL	1	2	3	4	5

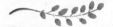 (1 = very low; 2 = low; 3 = moderate; 4 = high; 5 = very high)

MY MOOD

MORNING: _____

AFTERNOON: _____

EVENING: _____

ON MY MIND TODAY:

HOW I CARED FOR MYSELF TODAY

PHYSICAL: _____
_____

EMOTIONAL: _____
_____

MENTAL: _____
_____

PRACTICAL: _____
_____

SOCIAL: _____
_____

SPIRITUAL: _____
_____

TODAY I'M GRATEFUL FOR:

DATE: _____

LAST NIGHT'S SLEEP: _____HOURS _____MINUTES

QUALITY: _____

FOOD I ATE

MEAL 1

SNACKS & BEVERAGES

MEAL 2

MEAL 3

HYDRATION

◌ = 10 ounces of water

◌ ◌ ◌ ◌

◌ ◌ ◌ ◌

ACTIVITY	NOTES

ENERGY LEVEL 1   2   3   4   5

(1 = very low; 2 = low; 3 = moderate; 4 = high; 5 = very high)

MY MOOD

MORNING: _____

AFTERNOON: _____

EVENING: _____

ON MY MIND TODAY:

HOW I CARED FOR MYSELF TODAY

PHYSICAL: _____
_____

EMOTIONAL: _____
_____

MENTAL: _____
_____

PRACTICAL: _____
_____

SOCIAL: _____
_____

SPIRITUAL: _____
_____

TODAY I'M GRATEFUL FOR:

DATE: _____

LAST NIGHT'S SLEEP: _____HOURS _____ MINUTES

QUALITY: _____

FOOD I ATE

MEAL 1	SNACKS & BEVERAGES

MEAL 2

MEAL 3

HYDRATION

◊ = 10 ounces of water

◊ ◊ ◊ ◊

◊ ◊ ◊ ◊

ACTIVITY	NOTES

ENERGY LEVEL	1	2	3	4	5

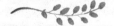

(1 = very low; 2 = low; 3 = moderate; 4 = high; 5 = very high)

MY MOOD

MORNING: _____

AFTERNOON: _____

EVENING: _____

ON MY MIND TODAY:

HOW I CARED FOR MYSELF TODAY

PHYSICAL: _____

_____

EMOTIONAL: _____

_____

MENTAL: _____

_____

PRACTICAL: _____

_____

SOCIAL: _____

_____

SPIRITUAL: _____

_____

TODAY I'M GRATEFUL FOR:

DATE: _____

LAST NIGHT'S SLEEP: _____ HOURS _____ MINUTES

QUALITY: _____

FOOD I ATE

MEAL 1	SNACKS & BEVERAGES

MEAL 2

MEAL 3

HYDRATION

⬥ = 10 ounces of water

⬥ ⬥ ⬥ ⬥

⬥ ⬥ ⬥ ⬥

ACTIVITY	NOTES

ENERGY LEVEL   1   2   3   4   5

(1 = very low; 2 = low; 3 = moderate; 4 = high; 5 = very high)

MY MOOD

MORNING: _____

AFTERNOON: _____

EVENING: _____

ON MY MIND TODAY:

HOW I CARED FOR MYSELF TODAY

PHYSICAL: _____

_____

EMOTIONAL: _____

_____

MENTAL: _____

_____

PRACTICAL: _____

_____

SOCIAL: _____

_____

SPIRITUAL: _____

_____

TODAY I'M GRATEFUL FOR:

DATE: _____

LAST NIGHT'S SLEEP: _____ HOURS _____ MINUTES

QUALITY: _____

FOOD I ATE

MEAL 1

MEAL 2

MEAL 3

SNACKS & BEVERAGES

HYDRATION
⬡ = 10 ounces of water

ACTIVITY	NOTES

ENERGY LEVEL	1	2	3	4	5

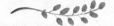

(1 = very low; 2 = low; 3 = moderate; 4 = high; 5 = very high)

MY MOOD

MORNING: _____

AFTERNOON: _____

EVENING: _____

ON MY MIND TODAY:

HOW I CARED FOR MYSELF TODAY

PHYSICAL: _____

_____

EMOTIONAL: _____

_____

MENTAL: _____

_____

PRACTICAL: _____

_____

SOCIAL: _____

_____

SPIRITUAL: _____

_____

TODAY I'M GRATEFUL FOR:

DATE: _____

LAST NIGHT'S SLEEP: _____ HOURS _____ MINUTES

QUALITY: _____

FOOD I ATE

MEAL 1

MEAL 2

MEAL 3

SNACKS & BEVERAGES

HYDRATION

◊ = 10 ounces of water

◊ ◊ ◊ ◊

◊ ◊ ◊ ◊

ACTIVITY

NOTES

| ENERGY LEVEL | 1 | 2 | 3 | 4 | 5 |

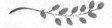

(1 = very low; 2 = low; 3 = moderate; 4 = high; 5 = very high)

MY MOOD

MORNING: _____

AFTERNOON: _____

EVENING: _____

ON MY MIND TODAY:

HOW I CARED FOR MYSELF TODAY

PHYSICAL: _____

_____

EMOTIONAL: _____

_____

MENTAL: _____

_____

PRACTICAL: _____

_____

SOCIAL: _____

_____

SPIRITUAL: _____

_____

TODAY I'M GRATEFUL FOR:

DATE: _____

LAST NIGHT'S SLEEP: _____ HOURS _____ MINUTES

QUALITY: _____

FOOD I ATE

MEAL 1	SNACKS & BEVERAGES
MEAL 2	
MEAL 3	**HYDRATION**
	◇ = 10 ounces of water
	◇ ◇ ◇ ◇
	◇ ◇ ◇ ◇

ACTIVITY	NOTES

ENERGY LEVEL 1   2   3   4   5

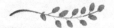

(1 = very low; 2 = low; 3 = moderate; 4 =.high; 5 = very high)

MY MOOD

MORNING: _____

AFTERNOON: _____

EVENING: _____

ON MY MIND TODAY:

HOW I CARED FOR MYSELF TODAY

PHYSICAL: _____
_____

EMOTIONAL: _____
_____

MENTAL: _____
_____

PRACTICAL: _____
_____

SOCIAL: _____
_____

SPIRITUAL: _____
_____

TODAY I'M GRATEFUL FOR:

DATE: _____

LAST NIGHT'S SLEEP: _____ HOURS _____ MINUTES

QUALITY: _____

FOOD I ATE

MEAL 1	SNACKS & BEVERAGES

MEAL 2	

MEAL 3	HYDRATION
	◊ = 10 ounces of water
	◊ ◊ ◊ ◊
	◊ ◊ ◊ ◊

ACTIVITY	NOTES

ENERGY LEVEL	1	2	3	4	5

(1 = very low; 2 = low; 3 = moderate; 4 = high; 5 = very high)

MY MOOD

MORNING: _____

AFTERNOON: _____

EVENING: _____

ON MY MIND TODAY:

HOW I CARED FOR MYSELF TODAY

PHYSICAL: _____

_____

EMOTIONAL: _____

_____

MENTAL: _____

_____

PRACTICAL: _____

_____

SOCIAL: _____

_____

SPIRITUAL: _____

_____

TODAY I'M GRATEFUL FOR:

DATE: _____

LAST NIGHT'S SLEEP: _____ HOURS _____ MINUTES

QUALITY: _____

FOOD I ATE

MEAL 1	SNACKS & BEVERAGES

MEAL 2

MEAL 3

HYDRATION

◊ = 10 ounces of water

◊ ◊ ◊ ◊
◊ ◊ ◊ ◊

ACTIVITY	NOTES

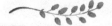

ENERGY LEVEL   1   2   3   4   5

(1 = very low; 2 = low; 3 = moderate; 4 = high; 5 = very high)

MY MOOD

MORNING: _____

AFTERNOON: _____

EVENING: _____

ON MY MIND TODAY:

HOW I CARED FOR MYSELF TODAY

PHYSICAL: _____
_____

EMOTIONAL: _____
_____

MENTAL: _____
_____

PRACTICAL: _____
_____

SOCIAL: _____
_____

SPIRITUAL: _____
_____

TODAY I'M GRATEFUL FOR:

DATE: _____

LAST NIGHT'S SLEEP: _____ HOURS _____ MINUTES

QUALITY: _____

FOOD I ATE

MEAL 1	SNACKS & BEVERAGES

MEAL 2

MEAL 3

HYDRATION

◌ = 10 ounces of water

◌ ◌ ◌ ◌

◌ ◌ ◌ ◌

ACTIVITY	NOTES

ENERGY LEVEL	1	2	3	4	5

(1 = very low; 2 = low; 3 = moderate; 4 = high; 5 = very high)

MY MOOD

MORNING: _____

AFTERNOON: _____

EVENING: _____

ON MY MIND TODAY:

HOW I CARED FOR MYSELF TODAY

PHYSICAL: _____

_____

EMOTIONAL: _____

_____

MENTAL: _____

_____

PRACTICAL: _____

_____

SOCIAL: _____

_____

SPIRITUAL: _____

_____

TODAY I'M GRATEFUL FOR:

DATE: _____

LAST NIGHT'S SLEEP: _____ HOURS _____ MINUTES

QUALITY: _____

FOOD I ATE

MEAL 1	SNACKS & BEVERAGES
MEAL 2	
MEAL 3	**HYDRATION**

HYDRATION

◊ = 10 ounces of water

◊ ◊ ◊ ◊

◊ ◊ ◊ ◊

ACTIVITY	NOTES

ENERGY LEVEL   1   2   3   4   5

(1 = very low; 2 = low; 3 = moderate; 4 = high; 5 = very high)

MY MOOD

MORNING: _____

AFTERNOON: _____

EVENING: _____

ON MY MIND TODAY:

HOW I CARED FOR MYSELF TODAY

PHYSICAL: _____
_____

EMOTIONAL: _____
_____

MENTAL: _____
_____

PRACTICAL: _____
_____

SOCIAL: _____
_____

SPIRITUAL: _____
_____

TODAY I'M GRATEFUL FOR:

DATE: _____

LAST NIGHT'S SLEEP: _____HOURS _____MINUTES

QUALITY: _____

FOOD I ATE

MEAL 1	SNACKS & BEVERAGES

MEAL 2	

MEAL 3	HYDRATION
	◊ = 10 ounces of water ◊ ◊ ◊ ◊ ◊ ◊ ◊ ◊

ACTIVITY	NOTES

ENERGY LEVEL	1	2	3	4	5

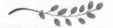

(1 = very low; 2 = low; 3 = moderate; 4 = high; 5 = very high)

MY MOOD

MORNING: _____

AFTERNOON: _____

EVENING: _____

ON MY MIND TODAY:

HOW I CARED FOR MYSELF TODAY

PHYSICAL: _____
_____

EMOTIONAL: _____
_____

MENTAL: _____
_____

PRACTICAL: _____
_____

SOCIAL: _____
_____

SPIRITUAL: _____
_____

TODAY I'M GRATEFUL FOR:

DATE: _____

LAST NIGHT'S SLEEP: _____ HOURS _____ MINUTES

QUALITY: _____

FOOD I ATE

MEAL 1	SNACKS & BEVERAGES

MEAL 2	

MEAL 3	HYDRATION
	◊ = 10 ounces of water

ACTIVITY	NOTES

ENERGY LEVEL	1	2	3	4	5

(1 = very low; 2 = low; 3 = moderate; 4 = high; 5 = very high)

MY MOOD

MORNING: _____

AFTERNOON: _____

EVENING: _____

ON MY MIND TODAY:

HOW I CARED FOR MYSELF TODAY

PHYSICAL: _____

_____

EMOTIONAL: _____

_____

MENTAL: _____

_____

PRACTICAL: _____

_____

SOCIAL: _____

_____

SPIRITUAL: _____

_____

TODAY I'M GRATEFUL FOR:

DATE: _____

LAST NIGHT'S SLEEP: _____ HOURS _____ MINUTES

QUALITY: _____

FOOD I ATE

MEAL 1	SNACKS & BEVERAGES

MEAL 2	

MEAL 3	HYDRATION
	⬧ = 10 ounces of water ⬧ ⬧ ⬧ ⬧ ⬧ ⬧ ⬧ ⬧

ACTIVITY	NOTES

ENERGY LEVEL	1	2	3	4	5

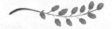

(1 = very low; 2 = low; 3 = moderate; 4 = high; 5 = very high)

MY MOOD

MORNING: _____

AFTERNOON: _____

EVENING: _____

ON MY MIND TODAY:

HOW I CARED FOR MYSELF TODAY

PHYSICAL: _____

_____

EMOTIONAL: _____

_____

MENTAL: _____

_____

PRACTICAL: _____

_____

SOCIAL: _____

_____

SPIRITUAL: _____

_____

TODAY I'M GRATEFUL FOR:

DATE:_____

LAST NIGHT'S SLEEP: _____ HOURS _____ MINUTES

QUALITY:_____

FOOD I ATE

MEAL 1

SNACKS & BEVERAGES

MEAL 2

MEAL 3

HYDRATION

◌ = 10 ounces of water

◌ ◌ ◌ ◌

◌ ◌ ◌ ◌

ACTIVITY

NOTES

| ENERGY LEVEL | 1 | 2 | 3 | 4 | 5 |

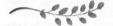

(1 = very low; 2 = low; 3 = moderate; 4 = high; 5 = very high)

MY MOOD

MORNING: _____

AFTERNOON: _____

EVENING: _____

ON MY MIND TODAY:

HOW I CARED FOR MYSELF TODAY

PHYSICAL: _____

_____

EMOTIONAL: _____

_____

MENTAL: _____

_____

PRACTICAL: _____

_____

SOCIAL: _____

_____

SPIRITUAL: _____

_____

TODAY I'M GRATEFUL FOR:

DATE: _____

LAST NIGHT'S SLEEP: _____ HOURS _____ MINUTES

QUALITY: _____

FOOD I ATE

MEAL 1

SNACKS & BEVERAGES

MEAL 2

MEAL 3

HYDRATION

◊ = 10 ounces of water

◊ ◊ ◊ ◊

◊ ◊ ◊ ◊

ACTIVITY	NOTES

ENERGY LEVEL   1   2   3   4   5

(1 = very low; 2 = low; 3 = moderate; 4 = high; 5 = very high)

MY MOOD

MORNING: _____

AFTERNOON: _____

EVENING: _____

ON MY MIND TODAY:

HOW I CARED FOR MYSELF TODAY

PHYSICAL: _____

_____

EMOTIONAL: _____

_____

MENTAL: _____

_____

PRACTICAL: _____

_____

SOCIAL: _____

_____

SPIRITUAL: _____

_____

TODAY I'M GRATEFUL FOR:

DATE: _____

LAST NIGHT'S SLEEP: _____ HOURS _____ MINUTES

QUALITY: _____

FOOD I ATE

MEAL 1

SNACKS & BEVERAGES

MEAL 2

MEAL 3

HYDRATION
⬦ = 10 ounces of water

⬦ ⬦ ⬦ ⬦

⬦ ⬦ ⬦ ⬦

ACTIVITY	NOTES

ENERGY LEVEL   1   2   3   4   5

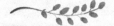

(1 = very low; 2 = low; 3 = moderate; 4 = high; 5 = very high)

MY MOOD

MORNING: _____

AFTERNOON: _____

EVENING: _____

ON MY MIND TODAY:

HOW I CARED FOR MYSELF TODAY

PHYSICAL: _____
_____

EMOTIONAL: _____
_____

MENTAL: _____
_____

PRACTICAL: _____
_____

SOCIAL: _____
_____

SPIRITUAL: _____
_____

TODAY I'M GRATEFUL FOR:

DATE: _____

LAST NIGHT'S SLEEP: _____ HOURS _____ MINUTES

QUALITY: _____

FOOD I ATE

MEAL 1	SNACKS & BEVERAGES
MEAL 2	
MEAL 3	**HYDRATION**
	⬦ = 10 ounces of water
	⬦ ⬦ ⬦ ⬦
	⬦ ⬦ ⬦ ⬦

ACTIVITY	NOTES

ENERGY LEVEL   1   2   3   4   5

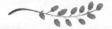

(1 = very low; 2 = low; 3 = moderate; 4 = high; 5 = very high)

MY MOOD

MORNING: _____

AFTERNOON: _____

EVENING: _____

ON MY MIND TODAY:

HOW I CARED FOR MYSELF TODAY

PHYSICAL: _____

_____

EMOTIONAL: _____

_____

MENTAL: _____

_____

PRACTICAL: _____

_____

SOCIAL: _____

_____

SPIRITUAL: _____

_____

TODAY I'M GRATEFUL FOR:

DATE: _____

LAST NIGHT'S SLEEP: _____HOURS _____MINUTES

QUALITY: _____

FOOD I ATE

MEAL 1	SNACKS & BEVERAGES

MEAL 2	

MEAL 3	HYDRATION
	◇ = 10 ounces of water

ACTIVITY	NOTES

ENERGY LEVEL	1	2	3	4	5

(1 = very low; 2 = low; 3 = moderate; 4 = high; 5 = very high)

MY MOOD

MORNING: _____

AFTERNOON: _____

EVENING: _____

ON MY MIND TODAY:

HOW I CARED FOR MYSELF TODAY

PHYSICAL: _____

_____

EMOTIONAL: _____

_____

MENTAL: _____

_____

PRACTICAL: _____

_____

SOCIAL: _____

_____

SPIRITUAL: _____

_____

TODAY I'M GRATEFUL FOR:

DATE: _____

LAST NIGHT'S SLEEP: _____ HOURS _____ MINUTES

QUALITY: _____

FOOD I ATE

MEAL 1

SNACKS & BEVERAGES

MEAL 2

MEAL 3

HYDRATION

◊ = 10 ounces of water

◊ ◊ ◊ ◊

◊ ◊ ◊ ◊

ACTIVITY	NOTES

ENERGY LEVEL	1	2	3	4	5

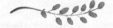

(1 = very low; 2 = low; 3 = moderate; 4 = high; 5 = very high)

MY MOOD

MORNING: _____

AFTERNOON: _____

EVENING: _____

ON MY MIND TODAY:

HOW I CARED FOR MYSELF TODAY

PHYSICAL: _____

_____

EMOTIONAL: _____

_____

MENTAL: _____

_____

PRACTICAL: _____

_____

SOCIAL: _____

_____

SPIRITUAL: _____

_____

TODAY I'M GRATEFUL FOR:

DATE: _____

LAST NIGHT'S SLEEP: _____ HOURS _____ MINUTES

QUALITY: _____

FOOD I ATE

MEAL 1

MEAL 2

MEAL 3

SNACKS & BEVERAGES

HYDRATION

⬥ = 10 ounces of water

⬥ ⬥ ⬥ ⬥

⬥ ⬥ ⬥ ⬥

ACTIVITY

NOTES

| ENERGY LEVEL | 1 | 2 | 3 | 4 | 5 |

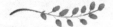

(1 = very low; 2 = low; 3 = moderate; 4 = high; 5 = very high)

MY MOOD

MORNING: _____

AFTERNOON: _____

EVENING: _____

ON MY MIND TODAY:

HOW I CARED FOR MYSELF TODAY

PHYSICAL: _____

_____

EMOTIONAL: _____

_____

MENTAL: _____

_____

PRACTICAL: _____

_____

SOCIAL: _____

_____

SPIRITUAL: _____

_____

TODAY I'M GRATEFUL FOR:

DATE: _____

LAST NIGHT'S SLEEP: _____ HOURS _____ MINUTES

QUALITY: _____

FOOD I ATE

MEAL 1	SNACKS & BEVERAGES

MEAL 2

MEAL 3

HYDRATION

◌ = 10 ounces of water

◌ ◌ ◌ ◌

◌ ◌ ◌ ◌

ACTIVITY	NOTES

ENERGY LEVEL	1	2	3	4	5

(1 = very low; 2 = low; 3 = moderate; 4 = high; 5 = very high)

MY MOOD

MORNING: _____

AFTERNOON: _____

EVENING: _____

ON MY MIND TODAY:

HOW I CARED FOR MYSELF TODAY

PHYSICAL: _____

_____

EMOTIONAL: _____

_____

MENTAL: _____

_____

PRACTICAL: _____

_____

SOCIAL: _____

_____

SPIRITUAL: _____

_____

TODAY I'M GRATEFUL FOR:

DATE: _____

LAST NIGHT'S SLEEP: _____ HOURS _____ MINUTES

QUALITY: _____

FOOD I ATE

MEAL 1	SNACKS & BEVERAGES
MEAL 2	
MEAL 3	**HYDRATION**
	◊ = 10 ounces of water
	◊ ◊ ◊ ◊
	◊ ◊ ◊ ◊

ACTIVITY	NOTES

ENERGY LEVEL   1   2   3   4   5

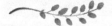

(1 = very low; 2 = low; 3 = moderate; 4 = high; 5 = very high)

MY MOOD

MORNING: _____

AFTERNOON: _____

EVENING: _____

ON MY MIND TODAY:

HOW I CARED FOR MYSELF TODAY

PHYSICAL: _____

_____

EMOTIONAL: _____

_____

MENTAL: _____

_____

PRACTICAL: _____

_____

SOCIAL: _____

_____

SPIRITUAL: _____

_____

TODAY I'M GRATEFUL FOR:

DATE: _____

LAST NIGHT'S SLEEP: _____ HOURS _____ MINUTES

QUALITY: _____

FOOD I ATE

MEAL 1	SNACKS & BEVERAGES
MEAL 2	
MEAL 3	**HYDRATION**
	⬦ = 10 ounces of water
	⬦ ⬦ ⬦ ⬦
	⬦ ⬦ ⬦ ⬦

ACTIVITY	NOTES

ENERGY LEVEL	1	2	3	4	5

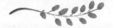

(1 = very low; 2 = low; 3 = moderate; 4 = high; 5 = very high)

MY MOOD

MORNING: _____

AFTERNOON: _____

EVENING: _____

ON MY MIND TODAY:

HOW I CARED FOR MYSELF TODAY

PHYSICAL: _____

_____

EMOTIONAL: _____

_____

MENTAL: _____

_____

PRACTICAL: _____

_____

SOCIAL: _____

_____

SPIRITUAL: _____

_____

TODAY I'M GRATEFUL FOR:

DATE: _____

LAST NIGHT'S SLEEP: _____ HOURS _____ MINUTES

QUALITY: _____

FOOD I ATE

MEAL 1

MEAL 2

MEAL 3

SNACKS & BEVERAGES

HYDRATION

◊ = 10 ounces of water

◊ ◊ ◊ ◊

◊ ◊ ◊ ◊

ACTIVITY	NOTES

ENERGY LEVEL 1 2 3 4 5

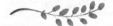

(1 = very low; 2 = low; 3 = moderate; 4 = high; 5 = very high)

MY MOOD

MORNING: _____

AFTERNOON: _____

EVENING: _____

ON MY MIND TODAY:

HOW I CARED FOR MYSELF TODAY

PHYSICAL: _____

_____

EMOTIONAL: _____

_____

MENTAL: _____

_____

PRACTICAL: _____

_____

SOCIAL: _____

_____

SPIRITUAL: _____

_____

TODAY I'M GRATEFUL FOR:

DATE: _____

LAST NIGHT'S SLEEP: _____ HOURS _____ MINUTES

QUALITY: _____

FOOD I ATE

MEAL 1	SNACKS & BEVERAGES

MEAL 2

MEAL 3

HYDRATION

◊ = 10 ounces of water

◊ ◊ ◊ ◊

◊ ◊ ◊ ◊

ACTIVITY	NOTES

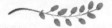

ENERGY LEVEL   1   2   3   4   5

(1 = very low; 2 = low; 3 = moderate; 4 = high; 5 = very high)

MY MOOD

MORNING: _____

AFTERNOON: _____

EVENING: _____

ON MY MIND TODAY:

HOW I CARED FOR MYSELF TODAY

PHYSICAL: _____

_____

EMOTIONAL: _____

_____

MENTAL: _____

_____

PRACTICAL: _____

_____

SOCIAL: _____

_____

SPIRITUAL: _____

_____

TODAY I'M GRATEFUL FOR:

DATE: _____

LAST NIGHT'S SLEEP: _____ HOURS _____ MINUTES

QUALITY: _____

FOOD I ATE

MEAL 1	SNACKS & BEVERAGES

MEAL 2

MEAL 3

HYDRATION
🜕 = 10 ounces of water
🜕 🜕 🜕 🜕
🜕 🜕 🜕 🜕

ACTIVITY	NOTES

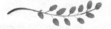

ENERGY LEVEL	1	2	3	4	5

(1 = very low; 2 = low; 3 = moderate; 4 = high; 5 = very high)

MY MOOD

MORNING: _____

AFTERNOON: _____

EVENING: _____

ON MY MIND TODAY:

HOW I CARED FOR MYSELF TODAY

PHYSICAL: _____
_____

EMOTIONAL: _____
_____

MENTAL: _____
_____

PRACTICAL: _____
_____

SOCIAL: _____
_____

SPIRITUAL: _____
_____

TODAY I'M GRATEFUL FOR:

DATE: _____

LAST NIGHT'S SLEEP: _____ HOURS _____ MINUTES

QUALITY: _____

FOOD I ATE

MEAL 1

SNACKS & BEVERAGES

MEAL 2

MEAL 3

HYDRATION
💧 = 10 ounces of water
💧 💧 💧 💧
💧 💧 💧 💧

ACTIVITY	NOTES

ENERGY LEVEL	1	2	3	4	5

(1 = very low; 2 = low; 3 = moderate; 4 = high; 5 = very high)

MY MOOD

MORNING: _____

AFTERNOON: _____

EVENING: _____

ON MY MIND TODAY:

HOW I CARED FOR MYSELF TODAY

PHYSICAL: _____

_____

EMOTIONAL: _____

_____

MENTAL: _____

_____

PRACTICAL: _____

_____

SOCIAL: _____

_____

SPIRITUAL: _____

_____

TODAY I'M GRATEFUL FOR:

DATE: _____

LAST NIGHT'S SLEEP: _____HOURS _____MINUTES

QUALITY: _____

FOOD I ATE

MEAL 1	SNACKS & BEVERAGES

MEAL 2

MEAL 3

HYDRATION

◊ = 10 ounces of water

◊ ◊ ◊ ◊
◊ ◊ ◊ ◊

ACTIVITY	NOTES

ENERGY LEVEL   1   2   3   4   5

(1 = very low; 2 = low; 3 = moderate; 4 = high; 5 = very high)

MY MOOD

MORNING: _____

AFTERNOON: _____

EVENING: _____

ON MY MIND TODAY:

HOW I CARED FOR MYSELF TODAY

PHYSICAL: _____

_____

EMOTIONAL: _____

_____

MENTAL: _____

_____

PRACTICAL: _____

_____

SOCIAL: _____

_____

SPIRITUAL: _____

_____

TODAY I'M GRATEFUL FOR:

DATE: _____

LAST NIGHT'S SLEEP: _____ HOURS _____ MINUTES

QUALITY: _____

FOOD I ATE

MEAL 1

MEAL 2

MEAL 3

SNACKS & BEVERAGES

HYDRATION

⬥ = 10 ounces of water

⬥ ⬥ ⬥ ⬥

⬥ ⬥ ⬥ ⬥

ACTIVITY

NOTES

ENERGY LEVEL   1   2   3   4   5

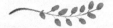 (1 = very low; 2 = low; 3 = moderate; 4 = high; 5 = very high)

MY MOOD

MORNING: _____

AFTERNOON: _____

EVENING: _____

ON MY MIND TODAY:

HOW I CARED FOR MYSELF TODAY

PHYSICAL: _____

_____

EMOTIONAL: _____

_____

MENTAL: _____

_____

PRACTICAL: _____

_____

SOCIAL: _____

_____

SPIRITUAL: _____

_____

TODAY I'M GRATEFUL FOR:

DATE: _____

LAST NIGHT'S SLEEP: _____ HOURS _____ MINUTES

QUALITY: _____

FOOD I ATE

MEAL 1

SNACKS & BEVERAGES

MEAL 2

MEAL 3

HYDRATION
◇ = 10 ounces of water

◇ ◇ ◇ ◇

◇ ◇ ◇ ◇

ACTIVITY	NOTES

ENERGY LEVEL	1	2	3	4	5

(1 = very low; 2 = low; 3 = moderate; 4 = high; 5 = very high)

MY MOOD

MORNING: _____

AFTERNOON: _____

EVENING: _____

ON MY MIND TODAY:

HOW I CARED FOR MYSELF TODAY

PHYSICAL: _____
_____

EMOTIONAL: _____
_____

MENTAL: _____
_____

PRACTICAL: _____
_____

SOCIAL: _____
_____

SPIRITUAL: _____
_____

TODAY I'M GRATEFUL FOR:

DATE: _____

LAST NIGHT'S SLEEP: _____ HOURS _____ MINUTES

QUALITY: _____

FOOD I ATE

MEAL 1	SNACKS & BEVERAGES

MEAL 2	

MEAL 3	HYDRATION
	💧 = 10 ounces of water

💧 💧 💧 💧

💧 💧 💧 💧

ACTIVITY	NOTES

ENERGY LEVEL   1   2   3   4   5

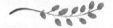

(1 = very low; 2 = low; 3 = moderate; 4 = high; 5 = very high)

MY MOOD

MORNING: _____

AFTERNOON: _____

EVENING: _____

ON MY MIND TODAY:

HOW I CARED FOR MYSELF TODAY

PHYSICAL: _____

_____

EMOTIONAL: _____

_____

MENTAL: _____

_____

PRACTICAL: _____

_____

SOCIAL: _____

_____

SPIRITUAL: _____

_____

TODAY I'M GRATEFUL FOR:

DATE: _____

LAST NIGHT'S SLEEP: _____ HOURS _____ MINUTES

QUALITY: _____

FOOD I ATE

MEAL 1	SNACKS & BEVERAGES
MEAL 2	
MEAL 3	**HYDRATION**
	◊ = 10 ounces of water
	◊ ◊ ◊ ◊
	◊ ◊ ◊ ◊

ACTIVITY	NOTES

ENERGY LEVEL	1	2	3	4	5

(1 = very low; 2 = low; 3 = moderate; 4 = high; 5 = very high)

MY MOOD

MORNING: _____

AFTERNOON: _____

EVENING: _____

ON MY MIND TODAY:

HOW I CARED FOR MYSELF TODAY

PHYSICAL: _____

_____

EMOTIONAL: _____

_____

MENTAL: _____

_____

PRACTICAL: _____

_____

SOCIAL: _____

_____

SPIRITUAL: _____

_____

TODAY I'M GRATEFUL FOR:

DATE: _____

LAST NIGHT'S SLEEP: _____HOURS _____MINUTES

QUALITY: _____

FOOD I ATE

MEAL 1

MEAL 2

MEAL 3

SNACKS & BEVERAGES

HYDRATION

◇ = 10 ounces of water

◇ ◇ ◇ ◇

◇ ◇ ◇ ◇

ACTIVITY	NOTES

ENERGY LEVEL	1	2	3	4	5

(1 = very low; 2 = low; 3 = moderate; 4 = high; 5 = very high)

MY MOOD

MORNING: _____

AFTERNOON: _____

EVENING: _____

ON MY MIND TODAY:

HOW I CARED FOR MYSELF TODAY

PHYSICAL: _____

_____

EMOTIONAL: _____

_____

MENTAL: _____

_____

PRACTICAL: _____

_____

SOCIAL: _____

_____

SPIRITUAL: _____

_____

TODAY I'M GRATEFUL FOR:

DATE: _____

LAST NIGHT'S SLEEP: _____ HOURS _____ MINUTES

QUALITY: _____

FOOD I ATE

MEAL 1	SNACKS & BEVERAGES
MEAL 2	
MEAL 3	**HYDRATION**
	◊ = 10 ounces of water
	◊ ◊ ◊ ◊
	◊ ◊ ◊ ◊

ACTIVITY	NOTES

ENERGY LEVEL	1	2	3	4	5

(1 = very low; 2 = low; 3 = moderate; 4 = high; 5 = very high)

MY MOOD

MORNING: _____

AFTERNOON: _____

EVENING: _____

ON MY MIND TODAY:

HOW I CARED FOR MYSELF TODAY

PHYSICAL: _____

_____

EMOTIONAL: _____

_____

MENTAL: _____

_____

PRACTICAL: _____

_____

SOCIAL: _____

_____

SPIRITUAL: _____

_____

TODAY I'M GRATEFUL FOR:

DATE: _____

LAST NIGHT'S SLEEP: _____ HOURS _____ MINUTES

QUALITY: _____

FOOD I ATE

MEAL 1	SNACKS & BEVERAGES

MEAL 2	

MEAL 3	HYDRATION
	◌ = 10 ounces of water
	◌ ◌ ◌ ◌
	◌ ◌ ◌ ◌

ACTIVITY	NOTES

ENERGY LEVEL	1	2	3	4	5

(1 = very low; 2 = low; 3 = moderate; 4 = high; 5 = very high)

MY MOOD

MORNING: _____

AFTERNOON: _____

EVENING: _____

ON MY MIND TODAY:

HOW I CARED FOR MYSELF TODAY

PHYSICAL: _____
_____

EMOTIONAL: _____
_____

MENTAL: _____
_____

PRACTICAL: _____
_____

SOCIAL: _____
_____

SPIRITUAL: _____
_____

TODAY I'M GRATEFUL FOR:

DATE: _____

LAST NIGHT'S SLEEP: _____ HOURS _____ MINUTES

QUALITY: _____

FOOD I ATE

MEAL 1	SNACKS & BEVERAGES

MEAL 2

MEAL 3

HYDRATION

◊ = 10 ounces of water

◊ ◊ ◊ ◊

◊ ◊ ◊ ◊

ACTIVITY	NOTES

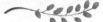

ENERGY LEVEL   1   2   3   4   5

(1 = very low; 2 = low; 3 = moderate; 4 = high; 5 = very high)

MY MOOD

MORNING: _____

AFTERNOON: _____

EVENING: _____

ON MY MIND TODAY:

HOW I CARED FOR MYSELF TODAY

PHYSICAL: _____

_____

EMOTIONAL: _____

_____

MENTAL: _____

_____

PRACTICAL: _____

_____

SOCIAL: _____

_____

SPIRITUAL: _____

_____

TODAY I'M GRATEFUL FOR:

DATE: _____

LAST NIGHT'S SLEEP: _____HOURS _____MINUTES

QUALITY: _____

FOOD I ATE

MEAL 1

SNACKS & BEVERAGES

MEAL 2

MEAL 3

HYDRATION

⬡ = 10 ounces of water

⬡ ⬡ ⬡ ⬡

⬡ ⬡ ⬡ ⬡

ACTIVITY	NOTES

ENERGY LEVEL	1	2	3	4	5

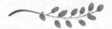

(1 = very low; 2 = low; 3 = moderate; 4 = high; 5 = very high)

MY MOOD

MORNING: _____

AFTERNOON: _____

EVENING: _____

ON MY MIND TODAY:

HOW I CARED FOR MYSELF TODAY

PHYSICAL: _____

_____

EMOTIONAL: _____

_____

MENTAL: _____

_____

PRACTICAL: _____

_____

SOCIAL: _____

_____

SPIRITUAL: _____

_____

TODAY I'M GRATEFUL FOR:

DATE: _____

LAST NIGHT'S SLEEP: _____HOURS _____MINUTES

QUALITY: _____

FOOD I ATE

MEAL 1	SNACKS & BEVERAGES

MEAL 2	

MEAL 3	HYDRATION
	◊ = 10 ounces of water
	◊ ◊ ◊ ◊
	◊ ◊ ◊ ◊

ACTIVITY	NOTES

ENERGY LEVEL	1	2	3	4	5

(1 = very low; 2 = low; 3 = moderate; 4 = high; 5 = very high)

MY MOOD

MORNING: _____

AFTERNOON: _____

EVENING: _____

ON MY MIND TODAY:

HOW I CARED FOR MYSELF TODAY

PHYSICAL: _____

_____

EMOTIONAL: _____

_____

MENTAL: _____

_____

PRACTICAL: _____

_____

SOCIAL: _____

_____

SPIRITUAL: _____

_____

TODAY I'M GRATEFUL FOR:

DATE: _____

LAST NIGHT'S SLEEP: _____ HOURS _____ MINUTES

QUALITY: _____

FOOD I ATE

MEAL 1	SNACKS & BEVERAGES
MEAL 2	
MEAL 3	**HYDRATION**
	⬦ = 10 ounces of water
	⬦ ⬦ ⬦ ⬦
	⬦ ⬦ ⬦ ⬦

ACTIVITY	NOTES

ENERGY LEVEL   1   2   3   4   5

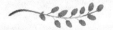

(1 = very low; 2 = low; 3 = moderate; 4 = high; 5 = very high)

MY MOOD

MORNING: _____

AFTERNOON: _____

EVENING: _____

ON MY MIND TODAY:

HOW I CARED FOR MYSELF TODAY

PHYSICAL: _____

_____

EMOTIONAL: _____

_____

MENTAL: _____

_____

PRACTICAL: _____

_____

SOCIAL: _____

_____

SPIRITUAL: _____

_____

TODAY I'M GRATEFUL FOR:

DATE: _____

LAST NIGHT'S SLEEP: _____ HOURS _____ MINUTES

QUALITY: _____

FOOD I ATE

MEAL 1	SNACKS & BEVERAGES

MEAL 2	

MEAL 3	HYDRATION
	⬦ = 10 ounces of water

ACTIVITY	NOTES

ENERGY LEVEL	1	2	3	4	5

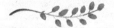

(1 = very low; 2 = low; 3 = moderate; 4 = high; 5 = very high)

MY MOOD

MORNING: _____

AFTERNOON: _____

EVENING: _____

ON MY MIND TODAY:

HOW I CARED FOR MYSELF TODAY

PHYSICAL: _____

_____

EMOTIONAL: _____

_____

MENTAL: _____

_____

PRACTICAL: _____

_____

SOCIAL: _____

_____

SPIRITUAL: _____

_____

TODAY I'M GRATEFUL FOR:

DATE: _____

LAST NIGHT'S SLEEP: _____ HOURS _____ MINUTES

QUALITY: _____

FOOD I ATE

MEAL 1

MEAL 2

MEAL 3

SNACKS & BEVERAGES

HYDRATION

◊ = 10 ounces of water

◊ ◊ ◊ ◊

◊ ◊ ◊ ◊

ACTIVITY

NOTES

ENERGY LEVEL

| 1 | 2 | 3 | 4 | 5 |

(1 = very low; 2 = low; 3 = moderate; 4 = high; 5 = very high)

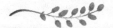

MY MOOD

MORNING: _____

AFTERNOON: _____

EVENING: _____

ON MY MIND TODAY:

HOW I CARED FOR MYSELF TODAY

PHYSICAL: _____
_____

EMOTIONAL: _____
_____

MENTAL: _____
_____

PRACTICAL: _____
_____

SOCIAL: _____
_____

SPIRITUAL: _____
_____

TODAY I'M GRATEFUL FOR:

DATE: _____

LAST NIGHT'S SLEEP: _____ HOURS _____ MINUTES

QUALITY: _____

FOOD I ATE

MEAL 1	SNACKS & BEVERAGES
MEAL 2	
MEAL 3	**HYDRATION**
	◊ = 10 ounces of water
	◊ ◊ ◊ ◊
	◊ ◊ ◊ ◊

ACTIVITY	NOTES

ENERGY LEVEL   1   2   3   4   5

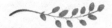

(1 = very low; 2 = low; 3 = moderate; 4 = high; 5 = very high)

MY MOOD

MORNING: _____

AFTERNOON: _____

EVENING: _____

ON MY MIND TODAY:

HOW I CARED FOR MYSELF TODAY

PHYSICAL: _____

_____

EMOTIONAL: _____

_____

MENTAL: _____

_____

PRACTICAL: _____

_____

SOCIAL: _____

_____

SPIRITUAL: _____

_____

TODAY I'M GRATEFUL FOR:

DATE: _____

LAST NIGHT'S SLEEP: _____ HOURS _____ MINUTES

QUALITY: _____

FOOD I ATE

MEAL 1	SNACKS & BEVERAGES
MEAL 2	
MEAL 3	**HYDRATION**
	◌ = 10 ounces of water
	◌ ◌ ◌ ◌
	◌ ◌ ◌ ◌

ACTIVITY	NOTES

ENERGY LEVEL	1	2	3	4	5

(1 = very low; 2 = low; 3 = moderate; 4 = high; 5 = very high)

MY MOOD

MORNING: _____

AFTERNOON: _____

EVENING: _____

> ON MY MIND TODAY:

HOW I CARED FOR MYSELF TODAY

PHYSICAL: _____
_____

EMOTIONAL: _____
_____

MENTAL: _____
_____

PRACTICAL: _____
_____

SOCIAL: _____
_____

SPIRITUAL: _____
_____

> TODAY I'M GRATEFUL FOR:

DATE: _____

LAST NIGHT'S SLEEP: _____ HOURS _____ MINUTES

QUALITY: _____

FOOD I ATE

MEAL 1	SNACKS & BEVERAGES
MEAL 2	
MEAL 3	**HYDRATION**
	◌ = 10 ounces of water
	◌ ◌ ◌ ◌
	◌ ◌ ◌ ◌

ACTIVITY	NOTES

ENERGY LEVEL 1   2   3   4   5

(1 = very low; 2 = low; 3 = moderate; 4 = high; 5 = very high)

MY MOOD

MORNING: _____

AFTERNOON: _____

EVENING: _____

ON MY MIND TODAY:

HOW I CARED FOR MYSELF TODAY

PHYSICAL: _____

_____

EMOTIONAL: _____

_____

MENTAL: _____

_____

PRACTICAL: _____

_____

SOCIAL: _____

_____

SPIRITUAL: _____

_____

TODAY I'M GRATEFUL FOR:

DATE: _____

LAST NIGHT'S SLEEP: _____ HOURS _____ MINUTES

QUALITY: _____

FOOD I ATE

MEAL 1	SNACKS & BEVERAGES
MEAL 2	
MEAL 3	**HYDRATION**
	◊ = 10 ounces of water
	◊ ◊ ◊ ◊
	◊ ◊ ◊ ◊

ACTIVITY	NOTES

ENERGY LEVEL	1	2	3	4	5

 (1 = very low; 2 = low; 3 = moderate; 4 = high; 5 = very high)

MY MOOD

MORNING: _____

AFTERNOON: _____

EVENING: _____

ON MY MIND TODAY:

HOW I CARED FOR MYSELF TODAY

PHYSICAL: _____

_____

EMOTIONAL: _____

_____

MENTAL: _____

_____

PRACTICAL: _____

_____

SOCIAL: _____

_____

SPIRITUAL: _____

_____

TODAY I'M GRATEFUL FOR:

DATE: _____

LAST NIGHT'S SLEEP: _____ HOURS _____ MINUTES

QUALITY: _____

FOOD I ATE

MEAL 1	SNACKS & BEVERAGES

MEAL 2	

MEAL 3	HYDRATION
	◇ = 10 ounces of water ◇ ◇ ◇ ◇ ◇ ◇ ◇ ◇

ACTIVITY	NOTES

ENERGY LEVEL	1	2	3	4	5

(1 = very low; 2 = low; 3 = moderate; 4 = high; 5 = very high)

MY MOOD

MORNING: _____

AFTERNOON: _____

EVENING: _____

ON MY MIND TODAY:

HOW I CARED FOR MYSELF TODAY

PHYSICAL: _____
_____

EMOTIONAL: _____
_____

MENTAL: _____
_____

PRACTICAL: _____
_____

SOCIAL: _____
_____

SPIRITUAL: _____
_____

TODAY I'M GRATEFUL FOR:

DATE: _____

LAST NIGHT'S SLEEP: _____HOURS _____MINUTES

QUALITY: _____

FOOD I ATE

MEAL 1

SNACKS & BEVERAGES

MEAL 2

MEAL 3

HYDRATION

◊ = 10 ounces of water

◊ ◊ ◊ ◊

◊ ◊ ◊ ◊

ACTIVITY

NOTES

ENERGY LEVEL   1   2   3   4   5

(1 = very low; 2 = low; 3 = moderate; 4 = high; 5 = very high)

MY MOOD

MORNING: _____

AFTERNOON: _____

EVENING: _____

ON MY MIND TODAY:

HOW I CARED FOR MYSELF TODAY

PHYSICAL: _____

_____

EMOTIONAL: _____

_____

MENTAL: _____

_____

PRACTICAL: _____

_____

SOCIAL: _____

_____

SPIRITUAL: _____

_____

TODAY I'M GRATEFUL FOR:

DATE: _____

LAST NIGHT'S SLEEP: _____ HOURS _____ MINUTES

QUALITY: _____

FOOD I ATE

MEAL 1

MEAL 2

MEAL 3

SNACKS & BEVERAGES

HYDRATION

◇ = 10 ounces of water

◇ ◇ ◇ ◇

◇ ◇ ◇ ◇

ACTIVITY

NOTES

ENERGY LEVEL   1   2   3   4   5

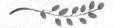

(1 = very low; 2 = low; 3 = moderate; 4 = high; 5 = very high)

MY MOOD

MORNING: _____

AFTERNOON: _____

EVENING: _____

ON MY MIND TODAY:

HOW I CARED FOR MYSELF TODAY

PHYSICAL: _____
_____

EMOTIONAL: _____
_____

MENTAL: _____
_____

PRACTICAL: _____
_____

SOCIAL: _____
_____

SPIRITUAL: _____
_____

TODAY I'M GRATEFUL FOR:

DATE: _____

LAST NIGHT'S SLEEP: _____ HOURS _____ MINUTES

QUALITY: _____

FOOD I ATE

MEAL 1	SNACKS & BEVERAGES
MEAL 2	
MEAL 3	**HYDRATION**
	⬤ = 10 ounces of water
	⬤ ⬤ ⬤ ⬤
	⬤ ⬤ ⬤ ⬤

ACTIVITY	NOTES

ENERGY LEVEL　　1　　　2　　　3　　　4　　　5

(1 = very low; 2 = low; 3 = moderate; 4 = high; 5 = very high)

MY MOOD

MORNING: _____

AFTERNOON: _____

EVENING: _____

ON MY MIND TODAY:

HOW I CARED FOR MYSELF TODAY

PHYSICAL: _____

_____

EMOTIONAL: _____

_____

MENTAL: _____

_____

PRACTICAL: _____

_____

SOCIAL: _____

_____

SPIRITUAL: _____

_____

TODAY I'M GRATEFUL FOR:

DATE: _____

LAST NIGHT'S SLEEP: _____ HOURS _____ MINUTES

QUALITY: _____

FOOD I ATE

MEAL 1

SNACKS & BEVERAGES

MEAL 2

MEAL 3

HYDRATION

◊ = 10 ounces of water

◊ ◊ ◊ ◊

◊ ◊ ◊ ◊

ACTIVITY

NOTES

ENERGY LEVEL   1   2   3   4   5

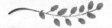

(1 = very low; 2 = low; 3 = moderate; 4 = high; 5 = very high)

MY MOOD

MORNING: _____

AFTERNOON: _____

EVENING: _____

ON MY MIND TODAY:

HOW I CARED FOR MYSELF TODAY

PHYSICAL: _____
_____

EMOTIONAL: _____
_____

MENTAL: _____
_____

PRACTICAL: _____
_____

SOCIAL: _____
_____

SPIRITUAL: _____
_____

TODAY I'M GRATEFUL FOR:

DATE: _____

LAST NIGHT'S SLEEP: _____HOURS _____MINUTES

QUALITY: _____

FOOD I ATE

MEAL 1	SNACKS & BEVERAGES

MEAL 2	

MEAL 3	HYDRATION
	◊ = 10 ounces of water
	◊ ◊ ◊ ◊
	◊ ◊ ◊ ◊

ACTIVITY	NOTES

ENERGY LEVEL	1	2	3	4	5

(1 = very low; 2 = low; 3 = moderate; 4 = high; 5 = very high)

MY MOOD

MORNING: _____

AFTERNOON: _____

EVENING: _____

ON MY MIND TODAY:

HOW I CARED FOR MYSELF TODAY

PHYSICAL: _____

_____

EMOTIONAL: _____

_____

MENTAL: _____

_____

PRACTICAL: _____

_____

SOCIAL: _____

_____

SPIRITUAL: _____

_____

TODAY I'M GRATEFUL FOR:

DATE: _____

LAST NIGHT'S SLEEP: _____ HOURS _____ MINUTES

QUALITY: _____

FOOD I ATE

MEAL 1	SNACKS & BEVERAGES
MEAL 2	
MEAL 3	**HYDRATION**
	⬭ = 10 ounces of water
	💧 💧 💧 💧
	💧 💧 💧 💧

ACTIVITY	NOTES

ENERGY LEVEL	1	2	3	4	5

(1 = very low; 2 = low; 3 = moderate; 4 = high; 5 = very high)

MY MOOD

MORNING: _____

AFTERNOON: _____

EVENING: _____

ON MY MIND TODAY:

HOW I CARED FOR MYSELF TODAY

PHYSICAL: _____

_____

EMOTIONAL: _____

_____

MENTAL: _____

_____

PRACTICAL: _____

_____

SOCIAL: _____

_____

SPIRITUAL: _____

_____

TODAY I'M GRATEFUL FOR:

DATE: _____

LAST NIGHT'S SLEEP: _____ HOURS _____ MINUTES

QUALITY: _____

FOOD I ATE

MEAL 1	SNACKS & BEVERAGES

MEAL 2	

MEAL 3	HYDRATION
	= 10 ounces of water

ACTIVITY	NOTES

ENERGY LEVEL	1	2	3	4	5

(1 = very low; 2 = low; 3 = moderate; 4 = high; 5 = very high)

MY MOOD

MORNING: _____

AFTERNOON: _____

EVENING: _____

ON MY MIND TODAY:

HOW I CARED FOR MYSELF TODAY

PHYSICAL: _____
_____

EMOTIONAL: _____
_____

MENTAL: _____
_____

PRACTICAL: _____
_____

SOCIAL: _____
_____

SPIRITUAL: _____
_____

TODAY I'M GRATEFUL FOR:

DATE: _____

LAST NIGHT'S SLEEP: _____HOURS _____MINUTES

QUALITY: _____

FOOD I ATE

MEAL 1	SNACKS & BEVERAGES
MEAL 2	
MEAL 3	**HYDRATION**
	⬦ = 10 ounces of water
	⬦ ⬦ ⬦ ⬦
	⬦ ⬦ ⬦ ⬦

ACTIVITY	NOTES

ENERGY LEVEL	1	2	3	4	5

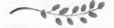

(1 = very low; 2 = low; 3 = moderate; 4 = high; 5 = very high)

MY MOOD

MORNING: _____

AFTERNOON: _____

EVENING: _____

ON MY MIND TODAY:

HOW I CARED FOR MYSELF TODAY

PHYSICAL: _____

_____

EMOTIONAL: _____

_____

MENTAL: _____

_____

PRACTICAL: _____

_____

SOCIAL: _____

_____

SPIRITUAL: _____

_____

TODAY I'M GRATEFUL FOR:

DATE: _____

LAST NIGHT'S SLEEP: _____ HOURS _____ MINUTES

QUALITY: _____

FOOD I ATE

MEAL 1	SNACKS & BEVERAGES
MEAL 2	
MEAL 3	**HYDRATION**

HYDRATION

◊ = 10 ounces of water

◊ ◊ ◊ ◊
◊ ◊ ◊ ◊

ACTIVITY	NOTES

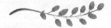

ENERGY LEVEL   1   2   3   4   5

(1 = very low; 2 = low; 3 = moderate; 4 = high; 5 = very high)

MY MOOD

MORNING: _____

AFTERNOON: _____

EVENING: _____

ON MY MIND TODAY:

HOW I CARED FOR MYSELF TODAY

PHYSICAL: _____

_____

EMOTIONAL: _____

_____

MENTAL: _____

_____

PRACTICAL: _____

_____

SOCIAL: _____

_____

SPIRITUAL: _____

_____

TODAY I'M GRATEFUL FOR:

DATE: _____

LAST NIGHT'S SLEEP: _____ HOURS _____ MINUTES

QUALITY: _____

FOOD I ATE

MEAL 1	SNACKS & BEVERAGES

MEAL 2	

MEAL 3	HYDRATION
	◇ = 10 ounces of water

◇ ◇ ◇ ◇

◇ ◇ ◇ ◇

ACTIVITY	NOTES

ENERGY LEVEL	1	2	3	4	5

(1 = very low; 2 = low; 3 = moderate; 4 = high; 5 = very high)

MY MOOD

MORNING: _____

AFTERNOON: _____

EVENING: _____

ON MY MIND TODAY:

HOW I CARED FOR MYSELF TODAY

PHYSICAL: _____

_____

EMOTIONAL: _____

_____

MENTAL: _____

_____

PRACTICAL: _____

_____

SOCIAL: _____

_____

SPIRITUAL: _____

_____

TODAY I'M GRATEFUL FOR:

DATE: _____

LAST NIGHT'S SLEEP: _____ HOURS _____ MINUTES

QUALITY: _____

FOOD I ATE

MEAL 1	SNACKS & BEVERAGES

MEAL 2	

MEAL 3	HYDRATION
	⬦ = 10 ounces of water
	⬦ ⬦ ⬦ ⬦
	⬦ ⬦ ⬦ ⬦

ACTIVITY	NOTES

ENERGY LEVEL	1	2	3	4	5

(1 = very low; 2 = low; 3 = moderate; 4 = high; 5 = very high)

MY MOOD

MORNING: _____

AFTERNOON: _____

EVENING: _____

ON MY MIND TODAY:

HOW I CARED FOR MYSELF TODAY

PHYSICAL: _____
_____

EMOTIONAL: _____
_____

MENTAL: _____
_____

PRACTICAL: _____
_____

SOCIAL: _____
_____

SPIRITUAL: _____
_____

TODAY I'M GRATEFUL FOR:

DATE: _____

LAST NIGHT'S SLEEP: _____ HOURS _____ MINUTES

QUALITY: _____

FOOD I ATE

MEAL 1

MEAL 2

MEAL 3

SNACKS & BEVERAGES

HYDRATION

◇ = 10 ounces of water

◇   ◇   ◇   ◇

◇   ◇   ◇   ◇

ACTIVITY	NOTES

ENERGY LEVEL	1	2	3	4	5

(1 = very low; 2 = low; 3 = moderate; 4 = high; 5 = very high)

MY MOOD

MORNING: _____

AFTERNOON: _____

EVENING: _____

ON MY MIND TODAY:

HOW I CARED FOR MYSELF TODAY

PHYSICAL: _____

_____

EMOTIONAL: _____

_____

MENTAL: _____

_____

PRACTICAL: _____

_____

SOCIAL: _____

_____

SPIRITUAL: _____

_____

TODAY I'M GRATEFUL FOR:

DATE: _____

LAST NIGHT'S SLEEP: _____ HOURS _____ MINUTES

QUALITY: _____

FOOD I ATE

MEAL 1	SNACKS & BEVERAGES

MEAL 2	

MEAL 3	HYDRATION
	△ = 10 ounces of water

ACTIVITY	NOTES

ENERGY LEVEL	1	2	3	4	5

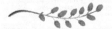

(1 = very low; 2 = low; 3 = moderate; 4 = high; 5 = very high)

MY MOOD

MORNING: _____

AFTERNOON: _____

EVENING: _____

ON MY MIND TODAY:

HOW I CARED FOR MYSELF TODAY

PHYSICAL: _____

_____

EMOTIONAL: _____

_____

MENTAL: _____

_____

PRACTICAL: _____

_____

SOCIAL: _____

_____

SPIRITUAL: _____

_____

TODAY I'M GRATEFUL FOR:

DATE: _____

LAST NIGHT'S SLEEP: _____ HOURS _____ MINUTES

QUALITY: _____

FOOD I ATE

MEAL 1	SNACKS & BEVERAGES

MEAL 2

MEAL 3

HYDRATION

◊ = 10 ounces of water

◊ ◊ ◊ ◊

◊ ◊ ◊ ◊

ACTIVITY	NOTES

ENERGY LEVEL   1   2   3   4   5

(1 = very low; 2 = low; 3 = moderate; 4 = high; 5 = very high)

MY MOOD

MORNING: _____

AFTERNOON: _____

EVENING: _____

ON MY MIND TODAY:

HOW I CARED FOR MYSELF TODAY

PHYSICAL: _____

_____

EMOTIONAL: _____

_____

MENTAL: _____

_____

PRACTICAL: _____

_____

SOCIAL: _____

_____

SPIRITUAL: _____

_____

TODAY I'M GRATEFUL FOR:

DATE: _____

LAST NIGHT'S SLEEP: _____HOURS _____MINUTES

QUALITY: _____

FOOD I ATE

MEAL 1	SNACKS & BEVERAGES

MEAL 2

MEAL 3	HYDRATION
	💧 = 10 ounces of water

ACTIVITY	NOTES

ENERGY LEVEL	1	2	3	4	5

(1 = very low; 2 = low; 3 = moderate; 4 = high; 5 = very high)

MY MOOD

MORNING: _____

AFTERNOON: _____

EVENING: _____

ON MY MIND TODAY:

HOW I CARED FOR MYSELF TODAY

PHYSICAL: _____

_____

EMOTIONAL: _____

_____

MENTAL: _____

_____

PRACTICAL: _____

_____

SOCIAL: _____

_____

SPIRITUAL: _____

_____

TODAY I'M GRATEFUL FOR:

DATE: _____

LAST NIGHT'S SLEEP: _____ HOURS _____ MINUTES

QUALITY: _____

FOOD I ATE

MEAL 1

SNACKS & BEVERAGES

MEAL 2

MEAL 3

HYDRATION
= 10 ounces of water

ACTIVITY	NOTES

ENERGY LEVEL	1	2	3	4	5

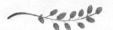 (1 = very low; 2 = low; 3 = moderate; 4 = high; 5 = very high)

MY MOOD

MORNING: _____

AFTERNOON: _____

EVENING: _____

ON MY MIND TODAY:

HOW I CARED FOR MYSELF TODAY

PHYSICAL: _____

_____

EMOTIONAL: _____

_____

MENTAL: _____

_____

PRACTICAL: _____

_____

SOCIAL: _____

_____

SPIRITUAL: _____

_____

TODAY I'M GRATEFUL FOR:

DATE: _____

LAST NIGHT'S SLEEP: _____ HOURS _____ MINUTES

QUALITY: _____

FOOD I ATE

MEAL 1	SNACKS & BEVERAGES

MEAL 2	

MEAL 3	HYDRATION

◌ = 10 ounces of water

ACTIVITY	NOTES

ENERGY LEVEL	1	2	3	4	5

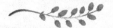

(1 = very low; 2 = low; 3 = moderate; 4 = high; 5 = very high)

MY MOOD

MORNING: _____

AFTERNOON: _____

EVENING: _____

ON MY MIND TODAY:

HOW I CARED FOR MYSELF TODAY

PHYSICAL: _____

_____

EMOTIONAL: _____

_____

MENTAL: _____

_____

PRACTICAL: _____

_____

SOCIAL: _____

_____

SPIRITUAL: _____

_____

TODAY I'M GRATEFUL FOR:

DATE: _____

LAST NIGHT'S SLEEP: _____ HOURS _____ MINUTES

QUALITY: _____

FOOD I ATE

MEAL 1	SNACKS & BEVERAGES
MEAL 2	
MEAL 3	**HYDRATION**
	⬭ = 10 ounces of water
	⬭ ⬭ ⬭ ⬭
	⬭ ⬭ ⬭ ⬭

ACTIVITY	NOTES

ENERGY LEVEL	1	2	3	4	5

(1 = very low; 2 = low; 3 = moderate; 4 = high; 5 = very high)

MY MOOD

MORNING: _____

AFTERNOON: _____

EVENING: _____

ON MY MIND TODAY:

HOW I CARED FOR MYSELF TODAY

PHYSICAL: _____

_____

EMOTIONAL: _____

_____

MENTAL: _____

_____

PRACTICAL: _____

_____

SOCIAL: _____

_____

SPIRITUAL: _____

_____

TODAY I'M GRATEFUL FOR:

DATE: _____

LAST NIGHT'S SLEEP: _____ HOURS _____ MINUTES

QUALITY: _____

FOOD I ATE

MEAL 1	SNACKS & BEVERAGES
MEAL 2	
MEAL 3	**HYDRATION**
	⬡ = 10 ounces of water
	💧 💧 💧 💧
	💧 💧 💧 💧

ACTIVITY	NOTES

ENERGY LEVEL	1	2	3	4	5

(1 = very low; 2 = low; 3 = moderate; 4 = high; 5 = very high)

MY MOOD

MORNING: _____

AFTERNOON: _____

EVENING: _____

ON MY MIND TODAY:

HOW I CARED FOR MYSELF TODAY

PHYSICAL: _____

_____

EMOTIONAL: _____

_____

MENTAL: _____

_____

PRACTICAL: _____

_____

SOCIAL: _____

_____

SPIRITUAL: _____

_____

TODAY I'M GRATEFUL FOR:

DATE: _____

LAST NIGHT'S SLEEP: _____ HOURS _____ MINUTES

QUALITY: _____

FOOD I ATE

MEAL 1	SNACKS & BEVERAGES
MEAL 2	
MEAL 3	**HYDRATION**

HYDRATION

◊ = 10 ounces of water

◊ ◊ ◊ ◊

◊ ◊ ◊ ◊

ACTIVITY	NOTES

ENERGY LEVEL   1   2   3   4   5

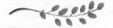

(1 = very low; 2 = low; 3 = moderate; 4 = high; 5 = very high)

MY MOOD

MORNING: _____

AFTERNOON: _____

EVENING: _____

ON MY MIND TODAY:

HOW I CARED FOR MYSELF TODAY

PHYSICAL: _____

_____

EMOTIONAL: _____

_____

MENTAL: _____

_____

PRACTICAL: _____

_____

SOCIAL: _____

_____

SPIRITUAL: _____

_____

TODAY I'M GRATEFUL FOR:

DATE: _____

LAST NIGHT'S SLEEP: _____ HOURS _____ MINUTES

QUALITY: _____

FOOD I ATE

MEAL 1	SNACKS & BEVERAGES
MEAL 2	
MEAL 3	**HYDRATION**
	💧 = 10 ounces of water

ACTIVITY	NOTES

ENERGY LEVEL	1	2	3	4	5

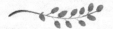

(1 = very low; 2 = low; 3 = moderate; 4 = high; 5 = very high)

MY MOOD

MORNING: _____

AFTERNOON: _____

EVENING: _____

ON MY MIND TODAY:

HOW I CARED FOR MYSELF TODAY

PHYSICAL: _____

_____

EMOTIONAL: _____

_____

MENTAL: _____

_____

PRACTICAL: _____

_____

SOCIAL: _____

_____

SPIRITUAL: _____

_____

TODAY I'M GRATEFUL FOR:

DATE: _____

LAST NIGHT'S SLEEP: _____ HOURS _____ MINUTES

QUALITY: _____

FOOD I ATE

MEAL 1	SNACKS & BEVERAGES
MEAL 2	
MEAL 3	**HYDRATION**
	◊ = 10 ounces of water
	◊ ◊ ◊ ◊
	◊ ◊ ◊ ◊

ACTIVITY	NOTES

ENERGY LEVEL	1	2	3	4	5

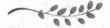

(1 = very low; 2 = low; 3 = moderate; 4 = high; 5 = very high)

MY MOOD

MORNING: _____

AFTERNOON: _____

EVENING: _____

ON MY MIND TODAY:

HOW I CARED FOR MYSELF TODAY

PHYSICAL: _____
_____

EMOTIONAL: _____
_____

MENTAL: _____
_____

PRACTICAL: _____
_____

SOCIAL: _____
_____

SPIRITUAL: _____
_____

TODAY I'M GRATEFUL FOR:

DATE: _____

LAST NIGHT'S SLEEP: _____HOURS _____MINUTES

QUALITY: _____

FOOD I ATE

MEAL 1

MEAL 2

MEAL 3

SNACKS & BEVERAGES

HYDRATION

💧 = 10 ounces of water

💧 💧 💧 💧

💧 💧 💧 💧

ACTIVITY

NOTES

ENERGY LEVEL

| 1 | 2 | 3 | 4 | 5 |

(1 = very low; 2 = low; 3 = moderate; 4 = high; 5 = very high)

MY MOOD

MORNING: _____

AFTERNOON: _____

EVENING: _____

ON MY MIND TODAY:

HOW I CARED FOR MYSELF TODAY

PHYSICAL: _____

_____

EMOTIONAL: _____

_____

MENTAL: _____

_____

PRACTICAL: _____

_____

SOCIAL: _____

_____

SPIRITUAL: _____

_____

TODAY I'M GRATEFUL FOR:

DATE: _____

LAST NIGHT'S SLEEP: _____ HOURS _____ MINUTES

QUALITY: _____

FOOD I ATE

MEAL 1	SNACKS & BEVERAGES
MEAL 2	
MEAL 3	**HYDRATION**
	⬤ = 10 ounces of water

ACTIVITY	NOTES

ENERGY LEVEL	1	2	3	4	5

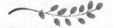

(1 = very low; 2 = low; 3 = moderate; 4 = high; 5 = very high)

MY MOOD

MORNING: _____

AFTERNOON: _____

EVENING: _____

ON MY MIND TODAY:

HOW I CARED FOR MYSELF TODAY

PHYSICAL: _____

_____

EMOTIONAL: _____

_____

MENTAL: _____

_____

PRACTICAL: _____

_____

SOCIAL: _____

_____

SPIRITUAL: _____

_____

TODAY I'M GRATEFUL FOR:

DATE: _____

LAST NIGHT'S SLEEP: _____ HOURS _____ MINUTES

QUALITY: _____

FOOD I ATE

MEAL 1	SNACKS & BEVERAGES
MEAL 2	
MEAL 3	**HYDRATION**
	◊ = 10 ounces of water
	◊ ◊ ◊ ◊
	◊ ◊ ◊ ◊

ACTIVITY	NOTES

ENERGY LEVEL	1	2	3	4	5

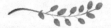

(1 = very low; 2 = low; 3 = moderate; 4 = high; 5 = very high)

MY MOOD

MORNING: _____

AFTERNOON: _____

EVENING: _____

ON MY MIND TODAY:

HOW I CARED FOR MYSELF TODAY

PHYSICAL: _____

_____

EMOTIONAL: _____

_____

MENTAL: _____

_____

PRACTICAL: _____

_____

SOCIAL: _____

_____

SPIRITUAL: _____

_____

TODAY I'M GRATEFUL FOR:

DATE: _____

LAST NIGHT'S SLEEP: _____ HOURS _____ MINUTES

QUALITY: _____

FOOD I ATE

MEAL 1

SNACKS & BEVERAGES

MEAL 2

MEAL 3

HYDRATION
⬤ = 10 ounces of water

ACTIVITY

NOTES

ENERGY LEVEL	1	2	3	4	5

(1 = very low; 2 = low; 3 = moderate; 4 = high; 5 = very high)

MY MOOD

MORNING: _____

AFTERNOON: _____

EVENING: _____

ON MY MIND TODAY:

HOW I CARED FOR MYSELF TODAY

PHYSICAL: _____

_____

EMOTIONAL: _____

_____

MENTAL: _____

_____

PRACTICAL: _____

_____

SOCIAL: _____

_____

SPIRITUAL: _____

_____

TODAY I'M GRATEFUL FOR:

DATE: _____

LAST NIGHT'S SLEEP: _____ HOURS _____ MINUTES

QUALITY: _____

FOOD I ATE

MEAL 1	SNACKS & BEVERAGES

MEAL 2	

MEAL 3	HYDRATION
	◇ = 10 ounces of water

◇ ◇ ◇ ◇

◇ ◇ ◇ ◇

ACTIVITY	NOTES

ENERGY LEVEL	1	2	3	4	5

(1 = very low; 2 = low; 3 = moderate; 4 = high; 5 = very high)

MY MOOD

MORNING: _____

AFTERNOON: _____

EVENING: _____

ON MY MIND TODAY:

HOW I CARED FOR MYSELF TODAY

PHYSICAL: _____

_____

EMOTIONAL: _____

_____

MENTAL: _____

_____

PRACTICAL: _____

_____

SOCIAL: _____

_____

SPIRITUAL: _____

_____

TODAY I'M GRATEFUL FOR:

DATE: _____

LAST NIGHT'S SLEEP: _____ HOURS _____ MINUTES

QUALITY: _____

FOOD I ATE

MEAL 1	SNACKS & BEVERAGES

MEAL 2	

MEAL 3	HYDRATION
	🜄 = 10 ounces of water

ACTIVITY	NOTES

ENERGY LEVEL	1	2	3	4	5

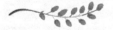

(1 = very low; 2 = low; 3 = moderate; 4 = high; 5 = very high)

MY MOOD

MORNING: _____

AFTERNOON: _____

EVENING: _____

ON MY MIND TODAY:

HOW I CARED FOR MYSELF TODAY

PHYSICAL: _____

_____

EMOTIONAL: _____

_____

MENTAL: _____

_____

PRACTICAL: _____

_____

SOCIAL: _____

_____

SPIRITUAL: _____

_____

TODAY I'M GRATEFUL FOR:

DATE: _____

LAST NIGHT'S SLEEP: _____ HOURS _____ MINUTES

QUALITY: _____

FOOD I ATE

MEAL 1	SNACKS & BEVERAGES
MEAL 2	
MEAL 3	**HYDRATION**
	◊ = 10 ounces of water
	◊ ◊ ◊ ◊
	◊ ◊ ◊ ◊

ACTIVITY	NOTES

ENERGY LEVEL	1	2	3	4	5

(1 = very low; 2 = low; 3 = moderate; 4 = high; 5 = very high)

MY MOOD

MORNING: _____

AFTERNOON: _____

EVENING: _____

ON MY MIND TODAY:

HOW I CARED FOR MYSELF TODAY

PHYSICAL: _____

_____

EMOTIONAL: _____

_____

MENTAL: _____

_____

PRACTICAL: _____

_____

SOCIAL: _____

_____

SPIRITUAL: _____

_____

TODAY I'M GRATEFUL FOR:

DATE: _____

LAST NIGHT'S SLEEP: _____ HOURS _____ MINUTES

QUALITY: _____

FOOD I ATE

MEAL 1

MEAL 2

MEAL 3

SNACKS & BEVERAGES

HYDRATION
◇ = 10 ounces of water

◇ ◇ ◇ ◇

◇ ◇ ◇ ◇

ACTIVITY	NOTES

ENERGY LEVEL	1	2	3	4	5

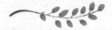

(1 = very low; 2 = low; 3 = moderate; 4 = high; 5 = very high)

MY MOOD

MORNING: _____

AFTERNOON: _____

EVENING: _____

ON MY MIND TODAY:

HOW I CARED FOR MYSELF TODAY

PHYSICAL: _____

_____

EMOTIONAL: _____

_____

MENTAL: _____

_____

PRACTICAL: _____

_____

SOCIAL: _____

_____

SPIRITUAL: _____

_____

TODAY I'M GRATEFUL FOR:

DATE: _____

LAST NIGHT'S SLEEP: _____ HOURS _____ MINUTES

QUALITY: _____

FOOD I ATE

MEAL 1	SNACKS & BEVERAGES

MEAL 2	

MEAL 3	HYDRATION
	⬨ = 10 ounces of water

⬨ ⬨ ⬨ ⬨

⬨ ⬨ ⬨ ⬨

ACTIVITY	NOTES

ENERGY LEVEL	1	2	3	4	5

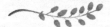

(1 = very low; 2 = low; 3 = moderate; 4 = high; 5 = very high)

MY MOOD

MORNING: _____

AFTERNOON: _____

EVENING: _____

ON MY MIND TODAY:

HOW I CARED FOR MYSELF TODAY

PHYSICAL: _____

_____

EMOTIONAL: _____

_____

MENTAL: _____

_____

PRACTICAL: _____

_____

SOCIAL: _____

_____

SPIRITUAL: _____

_____

TODAY I'M GRATEFUL FOR:

DATE: _____

LAST NIGHT'S SLEEP: _____ HOURS _____ MINUTES

QUALITY: _____

FOOD I ATE

MEAL 1

SNACKS & BEVERAGES

MEAL 2

MEAL 3

HYDRATION

◊ = 10 ounces of water

◊ ◊ ◊ ◊

◊ ◊ ◊ ◊

ACTIVITY

NOTES

| ENERGY LEVEL | 1 | 2 | 3 | 4 | 5 |

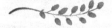

(1 = very low; 2 = low; 3 = moderate; 4 = high; 5 = very high)

MY MOOD

MORNING: _____

AFTERNOON: _____

EVENING: _____

ON MY MIND TODAY:

HOW I CARED FOR MYSELF TODAY

PHYSICAL: _____

_____

EMOTIONAL: _____

_____

MENTAL: _____

_____

PRACTICAL: _____

_____

SOCIAL: _____

_____

SPIRITUAL: _____

_____

TODAY I'M GRATEFUL FOR:

DATE: _____

LAST NIGHT'S SLEEP: _____ HOURS _____ MINUTES

QUALITY: _____

FOOD I ATE

MEAL 1	SNACKS & BEVERAGES

MEAL 2

MEAL 3	HYDRATION
	⬦ = 10 ounces of water

⬦ ⬦ ⬦ ⬦

⬦ ⬦ ⬦ ⬦

ACTIVITY	NOTES

ENERGY LEVEL	1	2	3	4	5

(1 = very low; 2 = low; 3 = moderate; 4 = high; 5 = very high)

MY MOOD

MORNING: _____

AFTERNOON: _____

EVENING: _____

ON MY MIND TODAY:

HOW I CARED FOR MYSELF TODAY

PHYSICAL: _____

_____

EMOTIONAL: _____

_____

MENTAL: _____

_____

PRACTICAL: _____

_____

SOCIAL: _____

_____

SPIRITUAL: _____

_____

TODAY I'M GRATEFUL FOR:

DATE: _____

LAST NIGHT'S SLEEP: _____ HOURS _____ MINUTES

QUALITY: _____

FOOD I ATE

MEAL 1	SNACKS & BEVERAGES
MEAL 2	
MEAL 3	**HYDRATION**
	◌ = 10 ounces of water
	◌ ◌ ◌ ◌
	◌ ◌ ◌ ◌

ACTIVITY	NOTES

ENERGY LEVEL	1	2	3	4	5

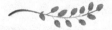

(1 = very low; 2 = low; 3 = moderate; 4 = high; 5 = very high)

MY MOOD

MORNING: _____

AFTERNOON: _____

EVENING: _____

ON MY MIND TODAY:

HOW I CARED FOR MYSELF TODAY

PHYSICAL: _____
_____

EMOTIONAL: _____
_____

MENTAL: _____
_____

PRACTICAL: _____
_____

SOCIAL: _____
_____

SPIRITUAL: _____
_____

TODAY I'M GRATEFUL FOR:

DATE: _____

LAST NIGHT'S SLEEP: _____ HOURS _____ MINUTES

QUALITY: _____

FOOD I ATE

MEAL 1	SNACKS & BEVERAGES
MEAL 2	
MEAL 3	**HYDRATION**
	⬦ = 10 ounces of water
	⬦ ⬦ ⬦ ⬦
	⬦ ⬦ ⬦ ⬦

ACTIVITY	NOTES

ENERGY LEVEL	1	2	3	4	5

(1 = very low; 2 = low; 3 = moderate; 4 = high; 5 = very high)

MY MOOD

MORNING: _____

AFTERNOON: _____

EVENING: _____

ON MY MIND TODAY:

HOW I CARED FOR MYSELF TODAY

PHYSICAL: _____

_____

EMOTIONAL: _____

_____

MENTAL: _____

_____

PRACTICAL: _____

_____

SOCIAL: _____

_____

SPIRITUAL: _____

_____

TODAY I'M GRATEFUL FOR:

DATE: _____

LAST NIGHT'S SLEEP: _____ HOURS _____ MINUTES

QUALITY: _____

FOOD I ATE

MEAL 1	SNACKS & BEVERAGES

MEAL 2

MEAL 3

HYDRATION

◊ = 10 ounces of water

◊ ◊ ◊ ◊

◊ ◊ ◊ ◊

ACTIVITY	NOTES

ENERGY LEVEL   1   2   3   4   5

(1 = very low; 2 = low; 3 = moderate; 4 = high; 5 = very high)

MY MOOD

MORNING: _____

AFTERNOON: _____

EVENING: _____

ON MY MIND TODAY:

HOW I CARED FOR MYSELF TODAY

PHYSICAL: _____

_____

EMOTIONAL: _____

_____

MENTAL: _____

_____

PRACTICAL: _____

_____

SOCIAL: _____

_____

SPIRITUAL: _____

_____

TODAY I'M GRATEFUL FOR:

DATE: _____

LAST NIGHT'S SLEEP: _____ HOURS _____ MINUTES

QUALITY: _____

FOOD I ATE

MEAL 1	SNACKS & BEVERAGES
MEAL 2	
MEAL 3	**HYDRATION**
	⬡ = 10 ounces of water
	💧 💧 💧 💧
	💧 💧 💧 💧

ACTIVITY	NOTES

ENERGY LEVEL	1	2	3	4	5

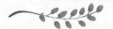

(1 = very low; 2 = low; 3 = moderate; 4 = high; 5 = very high)

MY MOOD

MORNING: _____

AFTERNOON: _____

EVENING: _____

ON MY MIND TODAY:

HOW I CARED FOR MYSELF TODAY

PHYSICAL: _____

_____

EMOTIONAL: _____

_____

MENTAL: _____

_____

PRACTICAL: _____

_____

SOCIAL: _____

_____

SPIRITUAL: _____

_____

TODAY I'M GRATEFUL FOR:

DATE: _____

LAST NIGHT'S SLEEP: _____ HOURS _____ MINUTES

QUALITY: _____

FOOD I ATE

MEAL 1	SNACKS & BEVERAGES

MEAL 2	

MEAL 3	HYDRATION
	◊ = 10 ounces of water
	◊ ◊ ◊ ◊
	◊ ◊ ◊ ◊

ACTIVITY	NOTES

ENERGY LEVEL	1	2	3	4	5

(1 = very low; 2 = low; 3 = moderate; 4 = high; 5 = very high)

MY MOOD

MORNING: _____

AFTERNOON: _____

EVENING: _____

ON MY MIND TODAY:

HOW I CARED FOR MYSELF TODAY

PHYSICAL: _____

_____

EMOTIONAL: _____

_____

MENTAL: _____

_____

PRACTICAL: _____

_____

SOCIAL: _____

_____

SPIRITUAL: _____

_____

TODAY I'M GRATEFUL FOR:

DATE: _____

LAST NIGHT'S SLEEP: _____HOURS _____ MINUTES

QUALITY: _____

FOOD I ATE

MEAL 1	SNACKS & BEVERAGES
MEAL 2	
MEAL 3	**HYDRATION**
	💧 = 10 ounces of water
	💧 💧 💧 💧
	💧 💧 💧 💧

ACTIVITY	NOTES

ENERGY LEVEL	1	2	3	4	5

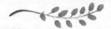

(1 = very low; 2 = low; 3 = moderate; 4 = high; 5 = very high)

MY MOOD

MORNING: _____

AFTERNOON: _____

EVENING: _____

ON MY MIND TODAY:

HOW I CARED FOR MYSELF TODAY

PHYSICAL: _____

_____

EMOTIONAL: _____

_____

MENTAL: _____

_____

PRACTICAL: _____

_____

SOCIAL: _____

_____

SPIRITUAL: _____

_____

TODAY I'M GRATEFUL FOR:

DATE: _____

LAST NIGHT'S SLEEP: _____HOURS _____MINUTES

QUALITY: _____

FOOD I ATE

MEAL 1	SNACKS & BEVERAGES

MEAL 2

MEAL 3

HYDRATION

◌ = 10 ounces of water

◌ ◌ ◌ ◌

◌ ◌ ◌ ◌

ACTIVITY	NOTES

ENERGY LEVEL	1	2	3	4	5

(1 = very low; 2 = low; 3 = moderate; 4 = high; 5 = very high)

MY MOOD

MORNING: _____

AFTERNOON: _____

EVENING: _____

ON MY MIND TODAY:

HOW I CARED FOR MYSELF TODAY

PHYSICAL: _____

_____

EMOTIONAL: _____

_____

MENTAL: _____

_____

PRACTICAL: _____

_____

SOCIAL: _____

_____

SPIRITUAL: _____

_____

TODAY I'M GRATEFUL FOR:

DATE: _____

LAST NIGHT'S SLEEP: _____HOURS _____MINUTES

QUALITY: _____

FOOD I ATE

MEAL 1	SNACKS & BEVERAGES

MEAL 2	

MEAL 3	HYDRATION
	△ = 10 ounces of water

ACTIVITY	NOTES

ENERGY LEVEL	1	2	3	4	5

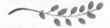

(1 = very low; 2 = low; 3 = moderate; 4 = high; 5 = very high)

MY MOOD

MORNING: _____

AFTERNOON: _____

EVENING: _____

ON MY MIND TODAY:

HOW I CARED FOR MYSELF TODAY

PHYSICAL: _____

_____

EMOTIONAL: _____

_____

MENTAL: _____

_____

PRACTICAL: _____

_____

SOCIAL: _____

_____

SPIRITUAL: _____

_____

TODAY I'M GRATEFUL FOR:

CPSIA information can be obtained
at www.ICGtesting.com
Printed in the USA
JSHW031225190122
22110JS00007B/193